All About
NUTRITION & AGING

By Laura Flynn R.N., B.N., M.B.A., in consultation with her nurse educator associates and physicians who assisted in contributing and editing.

Our thanks also to the fiollowing organization for their guidelines and use of educational material: Canada Food Guide 2010, New food Guide Pyramid US, American Heart Association, American Geriatric Society, Dieticians of Canada, American Dietetic Association and the best practice guidelines information from the Royal Nurses Association of Ontario.

ISBN No: 978 1 896616 64 3

©2011, 2017 Mediscript Communications Inc.

The publisher, Mediscript Communications Inc., acknowledges the financial support of the Government of Canada through the Canadian Book Fund for our publishing activities.

Nutrition & Elderly. Nutrition guidelines. Food guide for elderly. Food guide for older people.

www.mediscript.net

Printed in Canada

Book and Front Cover design by:
Brian Adamson, www.AdamsonGraphics.net

NU1002010

ALL ABOUT BOOKS

Trusted • Reliable • Certified

- 40+ titles available
- Comply with accreditation and regulatory bodies
- Suitable for caregivers, boomers with elderly parents, health workers, auxiliary health staff & patients
- Self study style with "test yourself" section
- Health On the Net (HON) certified
- A person or patient seeking information on nutrition and self care.

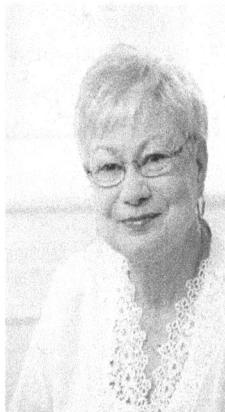

Some of our titles:

Alzheimers Disease	Arthritis	Multiple Sclerosis
Pain	Strokes	Elder Abuse
Falls Prevention	Incontinence	Nutrition & Aging
Personal Care	Positioning	Confusion
Transferring people	Care of the Back	Skin Care

For complete list of titles go to www.mediscript.net

Contact: 1 800 773 5088
Fax 1800 639 3186 • Email: mediscript30@yahoo.ca

CONTENTS

INTRODUCTION

This book provides basic, non controversial and trusted information that can help a wide spectrum of readers.

The primary objective of the information is to help a person provide effective quality care to a loved one or someone in his or her care.

After reading this material you will have greater confidence in your caregiving role and a better understanding of the role of nutrition in the overall care and well-being of older adults.

All the information is reliable and was written by a group of eminent nurse educators who ensured the information complies with best practice guidelines and satisfies the various accreditation and regulatory bodies. Because there is so much unreliable information on the internet, you can be assured the "All About" publications are HON (Health On the Net) certified.

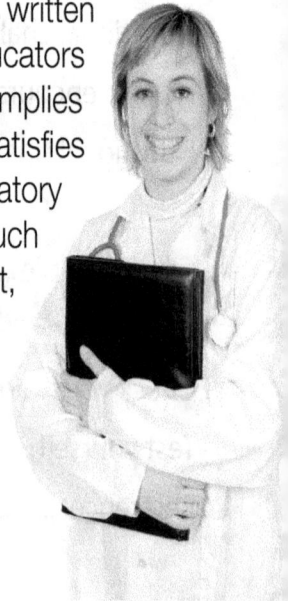

This book can be an invaluable aid to:

- A caregiver caring for a relative or friend
- A health worker seeking a reference aid
- Any person involved in health care wishing to expand his or her knowledge

---

SOMETHING TO THINK ABOUT...

Genius is one per cent inspiration,

ninety-nine per cent perspiration.

Thomas A. Edison

AN IMPORTANT MESSAGE
FROM THE PUBLISHER

Each person's treatment, advice, medical aids, physical therapy and other approaches to health care are unique and highly dependant upon the diagnosis and overall assessment by the medical team.

We emphasize therefore that the information within this book is not a substitute for the advice and treatment from a health care professional.

This book provides generic information concerning the issues around nutrition and older adults. Therefore, the publishers and authors disclaim any responsibility for any adverse effects resulting directly or indirectly from the suggestions contained within this book or from any misunderstanding of the content on the part of the reader.

HAVE YOU HEARD

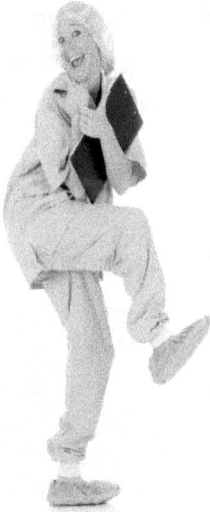

• "The most remarkable thing about my mother is that for 30 years she served the family nothing but leftovers. The original meal has never been found."

Sam Levinson

• "This recipe is certainly silly. It says to separate two eggs, but it doesn't say how far to separate them."

Gracie Allen

• "I've been on a constant diet for the last two decades. I've lost a total of 789 pounds. By all accounts, I should be hanging from a charm bracelet."

Erma Bombeck

HOW MUCH DO YOU KNOW?

It helps to figure out how much you know before you start. In this way you will have an idea as to the gaps in your knowledge prior to reading the content. Please circle to indicate the best answer. Remember, at this stage, you are not expected to know all the answers:

1. Which food item is the best source of protein?

A. Carrots

B. Brown rice

C. Apples

D. Cottage cheese

2. Which type of nutrient is most likely to cause gas?

A. Fiber

B. Protein

C. Fats

D. Carbohydrates

3. Which type of nutrient is available in both simple and complex forms?

A. Protein

B. Fiber

C. Carbohydrates

D. Vitamins and minerals

4. What is a common side effect of poor fluid intake in older adults?

A. Constipation

B. Gas

C. Heartburn

D. Incontinence

5. Which is the best strategy to reduce incontinence in older adults?

A. Avoid salty foods

B. Eat high acid foods

C. Decrease drinking fluids

D. Decrease drinking fluids after the evening meal

6. Which statement about food labels is most true?

A. Contents on the label are listed in order of the lowest to highest amount

B. Contents on the label are listed in order of the highest to lowest amount

C. Values on the labels are for all the food in the package

D. Labels are easy for older adults to read and understand

7. Why should older adults decrease caffeine in their diet?

A. It causes confusion

B. It is high in sodium

C. It causes stomach pains

D. It does not hydrate the body properly

ANSWERS

1. D. Of the four, cottage cheese is the best source of protein.

2. A. Fiber can cause gas, stomach pains, or diarrhea if added too quickly and in large amounts to a diet.

3. C. Carbohydrates come in two forms: simple and complex.

4. A. If older adults are afraid of becoming incontinent, they may avoid drinking enough water. This can cause constipation to occur.

5. D. It may help if older adults drink small frequent amounts throughout the day and not drink fluids after their evening meal.

6. B. Contents on the label are listed in order of the highest to lowest amount.

7. D. Caffeine increases thirst and does not hydrate the body properly.

WHY IS NUTRITION IMPORTANT
TO OLDER ADULTS?

Every person needs food to survive. The study of food and how it affects our bodies is called nutrition. Good nutrition is important for good health. Sometimes older people do not eat healthy foods. This can cause serious health problems such as obesity, under nutrition, or delayed recovery from illness. Food is a source of energy and nutrients. Nutrients are the substances in food that help build and maintain the cells of the body. As we age, we generally become less active. Our bodies, therefore, require less energy from food although we still need lots of nutrients. So the food we eat should be high in nutrients. This module tells you how to help older people get the nutrients that they need to maintain or enhance their quality of life.

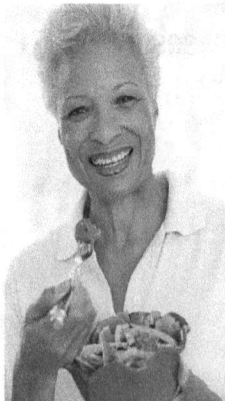

NUTRIENTS FOUND IN FOODS

The food and fluids we ingest provide important nutrients that our bodies require for longterm health. To get the nutrients you need, you must eat a balanced diet with all kinds of foods. Below are some of the nutrients found in the foods we eat:

Proteins

The best sources of protein are meat, milk, dairy products, and eggs. Plant foods provide protein if they are mixed with each other. Good protein mixes include beans with rice, lentils with bread, or vegetables with beans. Protein helps to build muscle and keep our immune systems healthy.

Older adults often lack protein in their diets. Here are some ways to increase protein intake:

- Add chopped, hard-cooked eggs to salads, vegetables and casseroles. If high cholesterol is a concern add only the egg white, not the yolk.

- Use milk to prepare hot cereal, soup, and puddings.

- Mix cottage cheese with, or use it to stuff, fruits and vegetables.

- Add cottage cheese to casseroles.

- Cook and use dried peas, legumes, beans, and tofu in soups or ethnic dishes.

- Add chopped meat or fish to salads, casseroles, and soups.

- Use peanut butter as a dip for raw fruits and vegetables.

- Spread peanut butter on sandwiches, toast, or crackers.

- Add nuts, seeds, and/or wheat germ to casseroles, breads, pancakes, and cookies.

- Sprinkle nuts, seeds, and/or wheat germ on fruit, cereal, ice cream, yogurt, and salads.

Fats

A diet high in fat can be harmful. The worst fats come from animal sources such as red meat and should only be eaten in very small amounts. However, there are "good" fats that come from fish and plant sources. These fats are called omega-3 fatty acids and are found in salmon, albacore tuna, sardines, lake trout, herring, and mackerel. Omega-3 fatty acids help protect the heart and decrease the amount of bad cholesterol in the blood. Other sources of "good" fat include tofu, soybeans, flaxseed, and vegetable oils. These sources contain a substance called alpha-linolenic acid, which can become omega-3 fatty acid in the body.

CONSIDER FOR A MOMENT ...

Consider your own diet. Is it high in
animal fats or in "good" fats like
those found in fish and plant sources?
Can you think of ways that you
can reduce the amount of harmful
fat in your diet?

Carbohydrates

Carbohydrates help to give us energy. Carbohydrates come in two forms: simple and complex Sources of simple carbohydrates include white breads, white rice, and sugar products. Simple carbohydrates are digested quickly. Complex carbohydrates take longer to digest but are healthier for us than simple carbohydrates. Complex carbohydrates include whole grain cereals, breads, and rice, fresh fruits, and fresh vegetables.

Fiber

Fiber is important to good health. Fiber helps to reduce constipation, lower cholesterol, and regulate blood sugar in diabetic clients. Good sources of fiber are fruits, vegetables, whole grain breads and cereals, and beans. Fiber can cause gas, stomach pains, or diarrhea if added too quickly and in large amounts to a diet. High fiber foods should be added gradually. Our bodies need time to adjust to a high fiber diet.

Vitamins and minerals

Vitamins and minerals are found in all kinds of foods and are very important for good health. Most people can get the vitamins and minerals they need if they follow "Canada's Food Guide" or the new Food Guide Pyramid (called MyPyramid) in the United States. Health Canada recommends that men and women over the age of 50 also take a daily vitamin D supplement of 10 µg (400 IU).

Other vitamins and minerals are available in pill form in cases where people do not or cannot get enough of these nutrients from their diets. No one should add vitamins and minerals to their diet until they talk to their doctors. Vitamins and minerals can be harmful if taken in very large amounts. Some of them can even interact with prescription medicines, over-the-counter medicines, and herbal preparations and cause bad side effects.

FOOD GUIDES

Canada and the United States (U. S.) use separate food guides. Both offer guidelines for healthy eating that are quite similar. Highlights of each guide are outlined below. If you live in the U. S., follow the new Food Guide Pyramid (MyPyramid). If you live in Canada, follow "Canada's Food Guide."

CANADA'S FOOD GUIDE

Canada's Food Guide makes recommendations for nutrition based on age and gender. Below are the recommended daily servings in Canada's food guide for adults 51 years of age and older.

Vegetables and fruit (fresh, frozen and canned)

Women need between 7-8 servings daily and men need 7-10 servings daily. Examples of one serving are:

- 1 cup of raw, leafy vegetables
- ½ cup of 100% juice
- ½ cup cooked vegetables
- 1 piece of medium-sized fruit such as a banana, apple, or orange

Grain products

Include breads, cereals, and pasta. Women need 6-7 servings a day. Men need 7-8 servings a day. Examples of one serving include:

- 1 slice of bread

- ¾ cup of hot cereal

- ½ cup of cold cereal

- ½ cup of cooked pasta

Grain Products | Vegetables & Fruit | Milk Products | Meat & Alternatives

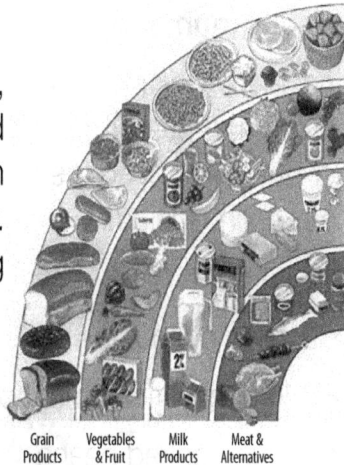

Milk products

Include milk, cheese, yogurt, and soy beverages. Women and men need 3 servings a day. It is recommended that adults drink 2 cups of skim, 1%, or 2% milk every day. Examples of one serving include:

- 1 cup powdered milk, mixed

- ¾ cup of yogurt

- 1 cup fortified soy beverage

Meat group

Includes meats, wild game, fish, poultry, eggs, beans, and peanut butter. Women need 2 servings per day. Men need 3 servings per day. Examples of one serving include:

- 2 eggs
- 2 Tbsp peanut butter
- 2 ½ ounces lean meat or poultry
- ¾ cup cooked beans

THE NEW FOOD GUIDE PYRAMID (United States)

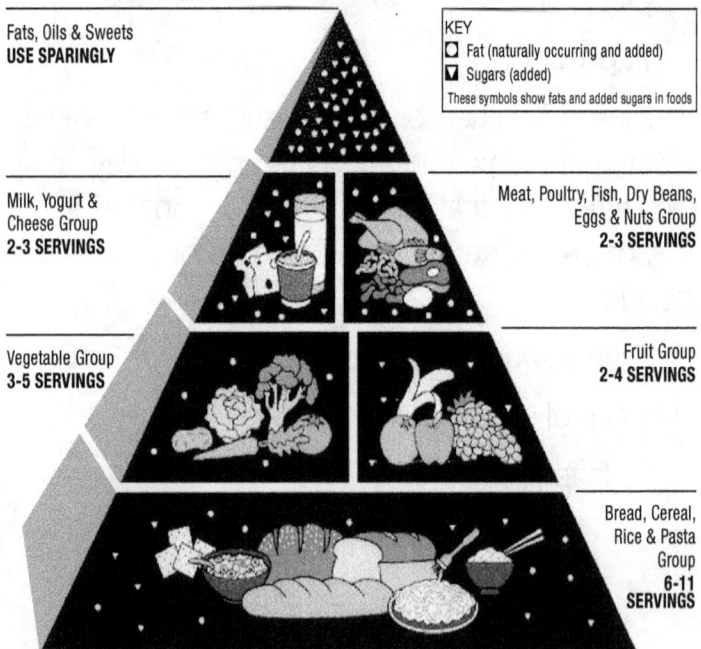

Fats, Oils & Sweets
USE SPARINGLY

KEY
☐ Fat (naturally occurring and added)
▼ Sugars (added)
These symbols show fats and added sugars in foods

Milk, Yogurt & Cheese Group
2-3 SERVINGS

Meat, Poultry, Fish, Dry Beans, Eggs & Nuts Group
2-3 SERVINGS

Vegetable Group
3-5 SERVINGS

Fruit Group
2-4 SERVINGS

Bread, Cereal, Rice & Pasta Group
6-11 SERVINGS

The new Food Guide Pyramid (MyPyramid) contains recommendations from the U. S. Department of Agriculture (USDA) for healthy eating. It contains six food groups and shows how many servings per day we should eat from each group. Here are the recommendations for adults:

Milk products

Include milk, cheese, and yogurt. Adults should eat 2-3 servings per day. Examples of one serving include:

1 cup of milk or yogurt

1 ½ ounces of natural cheese

2 ounces of process cheese

Fruits

Include both fruits and fruit juices. Adults should eat 2-4 servings per day. Examples of one serving include:

1 whole medium fruit

¼ cup dried fruit

½ cup canned fruit

½ to ¾ cup fruit juice

Vegetables

Include both vegetables and vegetable juice. Adults should eat 3-5 servings per day.

½ cup cooked vegetables

½ cup raw chopped vegetables

1 cup raw leafy vegetables

½ to ¾ cup vegetable juice

Meat group

Includes meat, eggs, fish, poultry, beans and nuts. Adults should eat 2-3 servings per day. Examples of one serving include:

2-3 ounces of cooked lean meat, poultry, or fish

2 eggs

7 ounces tofu

1 cup cooked legumes or dried beans or peas

½ cup nuts or seeds

Bread and cereals group

Include bread, cereal, rice and pasta. Adults should eat 6-11 servings per day. Examples of one serving include:

1 slice bread

1 medium muffin

1 cup cold cereal

½ cup cooked cereal

½ cup rice

½ cup pasta

Fats, oils, and sweets group

Include butter, sugar, gravy, salad dressing, and desserts. Foods in this group should be used sparingly.

NUTRITIONAL CHALLENGES

Many older adults have very little knowledge about healthy eating. Even when they know what foods will make them healthy, they may not always eat them. There are many reasons for this. Here are a few of the most common reasons.

Loneliness and isolation

The elderly may be lonely. Their children may live far away. They may be sad about the death of a spouse or other loved one. It is important to help older adults stay in contact with friends and family as much as possible. In fact, research shows that following the death of their husbands, women's appetites decrease as does their enjoyment of meals. Older adults often say that it is too much bother to cook for just themselves.

Loneliness can still exist even if the elderly live with family members or in long-term care settings. Elderly persons who live with adult children may be alone all day while these children are at work. Persons who live in group homes or long-term care settings may feel isolated from those they love and resent having to leave their own homes to live with strangers.

Poor fluid intake

Water is needed to help control body temperature, maintain skin integrity, and help bowel and bladder functioning. Older adults may not feel thirsty even when their bodies need water. Some elderly adults complain that they get too "full" when they drink a lot of fluid. Some are afraid of becoming incontinent if they drink too much. It may help if older adults drink small frequent amounts throughout the day and not drink fluids after their evening meal. This will help them to get the fluid they need and reduce the risk of incontinence.

Transportation, money, and health problems

Some older clients may not understand which foods are healthy for them. Many have trouble getting to a grocery store. Perhaps they no longer drive and do not have access to public transportation. They may not have enough money to use public transportation or to buy proper foods. Some elderly purchase canned soups and other products because they are less expensive and easy to prepare. They may buy microwave dinners for the same reasons. However, these foods are often high in salt and other non-healthy substances.

Dietary restrictions caused by culture and religion make it more challenging for older adults to follow a healthy diet. They may not be able to find the food they need or they may not be able to afford it. In fact, limited income may cause the elderly to decrease the amount of food they eat every day.

Older adults may have a variety of health problems. Conditions such as arthritis or stroke may make it difficult for them to shop, prepare and eat food. These problems may also make it hard to hold onto eating utensils. Chewing and swallowing may be affected. Many elderly clients are confused at times. All of these problems can interfere with their eating habits.

Many elderly adults take medicine because of chronic health problems. Drugs can cause appetite changes, decrease the taste of food, or cause nausea. It is important that older adults learn how to take their medicine so that it does not interfere with their nutrition. Some medicines should be taken on an empty stomach, while others should be taken with food. Some foods can cause bad side effects when taken with some medications. For example, grapefruit or grapefruit juice are not recommended while using some of the blood pressure, cholesterol, and heart medicines. Find out if your clients need to avoid certain foods or drink. If so, help them to do so.

Many older adults do not have the money or the interest to purchase properly fitting dentures or eyeglasses. Tooth decay as well as poorly fitting or missing dentures interfere with a person's ability to eat. Vision problems may make it difficult to prepare and eat healthy foods.

Digestion

Digestion is slower in older adults. This can cause heartburn, esophageal reflux, and gas. Elderly adults often do better eating small frequent meals instead of three large ones. And remember that when fiber is added to the diet, gas and stomach pains may occur. The elderly should add fiber slowly to the diet to avoid these problems.

Bowel and bladder function

Good nutrition is very important for proper bowel and bladder function. The large intestine (colon) moves more slowly than in younger adults. Bladder muscle may lose tone, causing incontinence. The diet must include fiber, water, and the right amounts of servings from the food groups to maintain bowel and bladder function. For example, if older adults are afraid of becoming incontinent, they may avoid drinking enough water. This can cause constipation to occur. Fiber found in fruits, vegetables, and whole grain foods also helps to keep the bowel normal. If older adults don't drink enough water they may not make enough urine. his can cause urinary tract infections.

Reading labels

Food labels are present on most prepackaged foods. They provide nutritional information so that consumers can make informed choices about the foods they buy. The list of ingredients on the label gives the contents in the order of highest amount to lowest amount. The values given on labels are for ONE serving only, not for the entire amount of food in the package. Older adults may need help to read these labels (they are sometimes written in tiny print) and to understand what they mean.

CONSIDER FOR A MOMENT ...
Select two packaged and two canned food items from your home. Estimate which ingredients are present in the highest amounts ineach of the four food items.
Then read the labels.
How close were your estimates?

Handling and storing food

Older adults may not know how to safely handle and store food. Here are some tips for doing so:

1. Refrigerate or freeze all perishable foods.

2. Always thaw food in the refrigerator, NEVER at room temperature.

3. Always wash hands, utensils, cutting boards and other work surfaces after they touch raw meat or poultry.

4. Never leave perishable foods out of the refrigerator over 2 hours.

5. Never eat raw or under-cooked meat, poultry, fish, or eggs.

HOW TO ENCOURAGE HEALTHY EATING

Loneliness and isolation

Resources are available to help reduce the loneliness and isolation of the elderly, especially at mealtime. Many healthcare facilities have a volunteer department that can provide trained volunteers to help set up meal trays and feed clients while providing company and support. In the community, organizations such as adult day care centers and senior citizen centers can provide companionship and activities as well as healthy meals. "Meals on Wheels" programs deliver low priced, nutritious meals to the homes of the elderly. Encourage family or friends to arrange visits at mealtime. Some older clients in the community may wish to take turns preparing and sharing meals with friends.

Health care agencies need to work with colleges and universities to help promote student projects that encourage good nutrition. Student clinicians could become involved in visiting with clients as they eat and also teaching them about good nutrition. The elderly living in their homes, hospitals or long term care settings could benefit immensely from student nutrition projects.

Fluid intake

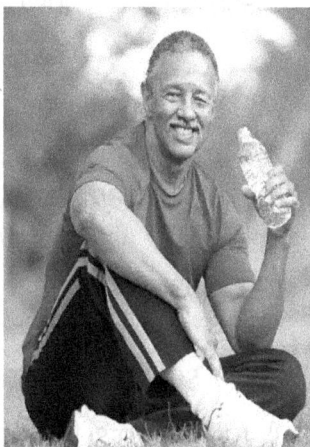

Teach older adults to avoid drinks that contain caffeine and alcohol. These increase thirst and do not hydrate the body properly. Offer water at frequent times throughout the day. The elderly may find it easier to drink small amounts of water throughout the day rather than several large glasses. To reduce incontinence, fluids should not be taken after the evening meal.

Dry, bulky, spicy, salty, or very acidic foods should be avoided. These increase thirst and are often high in sodium. They also interfere with hydration. If thirst persists late into the evening clients may eat sugarless hard candy or chewing gum to reduce thirst. However, clients who have dementia or trouble swallowing should not chew gum or eat hard candy. Petroleum jelly (Vaseline) may be applied to the lips to soothe dry, cracked lips.

Transportation, money, and health problems

- Make a list of public transportation options (e.g. buses, taxi cabs) that offer discounts to older clients with mobility problems. Give copies of these lists to your clients who live at home and also to their families as needed.

- Make a list of ways to help elderly adults save money on food. For example, using coupons and reading advertisements about food sales would help older adults save money. Refer your clients to organizations that can help them budget their money. Examples include senior citizen centers, social services, and agencies on aging.

- Assess clients for properly fitting dentures, tooth and gum problems, and eyeglasses that are the right prescription. Keep a list of dentists and eye doctors who specialize in treating the elderly and who may offer discounts on their services for older adults.

- Help clients and their families keep an up-to-date list of ALL medications the older client takes, including prescription drugs, over-the-counter medications, vitamin and mineral supplements, and herbal supplements. They should take this list with them whenever they have a doctor's appointment. Teach them to ask their doctors about any side effects or interactions that might occur. Teach them to ask their doctors about any foods they should avoid because of the medicines they take.

Digestion

Explain to your clients that as they age, it takes longer to digest food. Here are some tips to help them with their digestion:

- Avoid salty and highly spicy foods.

- Eat foods that are high in acid (e.g. tomatoes) in small amounts.

- When adding high-fiber foods to the diet, be aware that these foods can cause gas and stomach pains. Add high-fiber foods gradually to the diet.

- Avoid foods that are high in salt (sodium) such as canned soups and microwave dinners. Encourage them to avoid salting their food at the table.

- Avoid foods that are high in saturated, animal fats (e.g. red meat, butter) or eat them only in rather small amounts.

- Help clients learn to read food labels and make decisions based on the content of foods.

- Eat small frequent meals spaced throughout the day instead of three big meals.

- Older adults who can't or won't eat may benefit from eating or drinking high-calorie, nutrient-rich supplements. They should consult their doctors about which supplements are best for them.

Bowel and bladder control

- Avoid drinking large amounts of fluids after the evening meal.

- Clients need to understand that they should drink plenty of water or other non-caffeine beverages every day to have good bowel and bladder health. Drink small amounts of fluid instead of large glasses that may make older adults feel "full" and uncomfortable.

- Clients need to understand that water intake is important to prevent constipation.

NUTRITIONAL TIPS FOR CAREGIVERS

Making sure tha elderly people receive proper nutrition can be a challenge. As a caregiver or healthworker, you can be very busy and it takes time and patience to help older people eat. But remember how important it is to good health to eat healthy foods and drink enough fluids.

Sometimes older people and family members can forget just how important proper nutrition can be, so it is up to you to show them how to enjoy meals while still getting the proper amount of nutrients. Here are some ways to do both:

- Check on the person's nutritional status frequently. Older adults can develop eating problems quickly. If you suspect that an older adult has a nutrition problem, take action immediately.

- If you are a healthworker do not take do not take "breaks" or meals when clients are eating their meals. This will help to make sure enough staff members are available to help clients eat. Work with your fellow healthcare workers to schedule your breaks and meals so they don't interfere with helping your clients.

- Make sure commodes, urinals, and trash are removed from the person's view when he or she is eating. No one wants to look at commodes, urinals, or trash when eating.

- Consider the eating area. Is it crowded, noisy, unpleasant? Perhaps your client would prefer to eat alone or in a quiet area with a friend. If your client is confused, a noisy environment may result in agitation. The client may be more confused and not able to focus on the meal.

- If appropriate, ensure that pain medication and pills to prevent vomiting are given before meals.

- Assist elderly people to sit up while eating. Avoid feeding person in bed, if possible. Help them to sit in a comfortable chair.

- Do not schedule visits or procedures during meal time.

- Assist elderly people to wash their hands before meals.

- Make sure elderly peoples' dentures are in place and eyeglasses are on before mealtime.

- Offer mouth care before and after meals.

- Encourage elderly people to drink water often throughout the day (unless the physician has ordered that fluids be restricted).

- If the older person is not available when meals are served, keep their trays warm. No one likes to eat cold food!

- Help your elderly people and families learn about healthy eating.

- Find out what your client likes to eat. Pass that information on to the nutritionist if a nutritionist is involved in your client's care.

- When able, encourage family members to help feed clients and/or to sit with them at meal times.

- Keep a careful record of the older person's height and weight. Changes in weight may indicate too many or too few calories and nutrients. Remember that older adults may actually decrease in height as they age.

- Oral supplements should be given between meals. They should not take the place of regular meals and should not be served within the hour before a meal.

- Find out about the elderly person's favorite foods. Ensure that some of those are included in the diet.

- When you are feeding someone, do not mix all the foods together. Offer one food at a time.

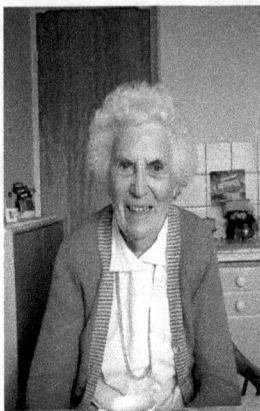

CASE EXAMPLE

Mrs. Rowe is seventy-six years old and lives alone in her own home. Fiercely independent, she has been able to function quite well on her own since her husband's death over ten years ago. Mrs. Rowe is well known in her neighborhood for her friendly manner, her ready smile, and her daily walks with her collie, Rex.

Over the past few months, Mrs. Rowe has become much more frail. She can't seem to manage the long walks anymore, has been skipping meals, and has lost a few pounds. Her doctor recently examined Mrs. Rowe and could find nothing medically wrong. Mrs. Rowe confided to her doctor at that time that she had lost interest in shopping, cooking, and eating.

Mrs. Rowe's family are concerned about her increasing frailty and poor diet. They have hired you to visit four times a week. They would like to see an improvement in their mother's diet and have asked you to develop a meal plan for her breakfast, lunch, and supper. The plan would have to include a variety of healthy foods that would provide Mrs. Rowe with a balanced diet.

Using highlights from the appropriate food guide, develop a healthy meal plan with at least three options for breakfast, lunch, and supper. (When preparing a meal plan for your clients, you would most likely need to develop more than three options for each meal.)

YOUR ANSWERS TO CASE EXAMPLE

SUGGESTED ANSWER TO CASE EXAMPLE

The meal plan outlined below assumes that Mrs. Rowe has no particular food restrictions or dislikes. The suggested meals are inexpensive, healthy, and easy to prepare.

Day One

Breakfast - Poached egg, whole grain toast, orange juice, and fruit (e.g. banana, prunes, etc.)

Lunch - Vegetable soup, chicken sandwich on whole gain bread, an apple, and a glass of skim milk

Snack - Yogurt and a piece of fresh fruit (e.g. banana, peach, apple, etc.)

Supper - Spaghetti with meat sauce, salad made with lettuce and raw vegetables (e.g. tomatoes, cucumbers, broccoli, etc.), and a glass of skim milk

Day Two

Breakfast - Hot cereal with a banana, skim milk, orange or apple juice

Lunch - Macaroni and cheese with tomato slices, skim milk, and fruit

Snack - Fruit salad and whole wheat crackers

Supper - Baked fish, potato, green beans, slice of whole grain bread, skim milk, and a piece of fresh fruit

Day Three

Breakfast - Pancakes, skim milk, and applesauce

Lunch - Whole grain bread with peanut butter, banana, and skim milk

Snack - Cheese and whole wheat crackers and a piece of fresh fruit

Supper - Stir-fry beef or chicken with a variety of fresh or frozen vegetables served over rice or pasta, fruit cocktail, and skim milk.

Good nutrition is important to persons of all ages. Older adults have particular nutritional challenges that can result in a poorer quality of life. Healthcare workers can use many strategies to promote healthy eating for older adults.

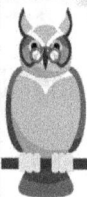

CHECK YOUR KNOWLEDGE

1. What major food groups are needed for a healthy diet? (Refer to the appropriate food guide.)

2. What is the recommended number of servings of each group per day?

3. List four nutritional challenges facing older adults.

4. Identify four strategies that you can use to encourage older adults to follow a healthy diet.

TEST YOURSELF

Please circle to indicate the best answer:

1. Which nutrient needs to be added to the diet slowly?

A. Protein

B. Fiber

C. Carbohydrates

D. Vitamins and minerals

2. How do older adults benefit from an adequate fluid intake?

A. Provides extra energy

B. Important source of fiber

C. Helps bowel and bladder function

D. Provides vitamins

3. What is a benefit of eating small frequent meals?

A. Prevents gas

B. Prevents diarrhea

C. Provides more protein

D. Protects against incontinence

4. Which statement about older adults is most true?

A. Three large meals a day are best

B. Older adults don't like to eat alone

C. Older adults like to eat in a busy, noisy environment

D. Older adults prefer to have all their food mixed together at meal time

5. What is a benefit of protein in the diet?

A. Improves digestion

B. Improves the taste of food

C. Lowers cholesterol

D. Keeps the immune system healthy

6. What strategy would be most helpful to promote digestion among older adults?

A. Take multivitamins

B. Eat lots of foods high in acid

C. Eat spicy foods

D. Eat small, frequent meals

7. Which food would be best to include in a meal plan for an older adult?

A. Skim milk because it's low in fat

B. White bread because it is digested quickly

C. Butter because it is an important source of fat

D. White rice because it is an important source of carbohydrates

ANSWERS

1. B. Fiber can cause gas, stomach pains, or diarrhea if added too quickly and in large amounts to a diet.

2. C. Water is needed to help control body temperature, maintain skin integrity, and help bowel and bladder functioning.

3. A. Digestion is slower in older adults. This can cause heartburn, esophageal reflux, and gas.

4. B. Resources are available to help reduce the loneliness and isolation of the elderly, especially at mealtime. Encourage family or friends to arrange visits at mealtime.

5. D. Protein helps to build muscle and keep our immune systems healthy.

6. D. Elderly adults often do better eating small frequent meals instead of three large ones.

7. A. Both Canada's Food Guide and MyPyramid recommend skim milk for older adults because of its low fat content.

REFERENCES

American Family Physician. (2007). Medicine interactions with grapefruit: What you should know. Retrieved April 27, 2007 www.aafp.org/afp/20060815/611ph.html.

American Heart Association. (2007). Fish and omega-3 fatty acids. Retrieved April 25, 2007 www.americanheart.org.

Avillion, A. E. (2004). Age-specific care training handbook for nurses and clinical care staff. Marblehead, MASS: hcPro.

DiMaria-Ghalili, R. A., & Amella, E. (2005). Nutrition in older adults: Intervention and assessment can help curb the growing threat of malnutrition. AJN, 105(3), 40-50.

Disabled World. (2007). The old and the new food pyramid. Retrieved April 23 http://www.disabled-world.com/artman/publish/food_pyramid.shtml

Health Canada. (2007). Eating well with Canada's food guide. Retrieved April 23, 2007 www.hc-sc.gc.ca/fn-an/pubs/fnim-pnim/index_e.html

Johnson, R. M. (2005). A case study in service-learning: A community nutrition food drive - neighbors helping neighbors. Topics in Clinical Nutrition, 20(4), 351-356.

Pray, W. S. (2006). The health benefits of fiber. Retrieved April 25, 2007"www.medscape.com.

U. S. Department of Agriculture. (2006). Safe food handling. Retrieved April 23, 2007 www.fsis.usda.gov/Fact_Sheets/Seniors_need_Wisdom_on_Food_Safety/index.asp.

U. S. Food and Drug Administration. (2004). How to understand and use the nutrition facts label. Retrieved on April 23, 2007 http://www.cfsan.fda.gov/~dms/foodlab.html

Wardlaw, G., & Insel, P. (1996). Perspectives in nutrition (3rd ed.). St. Louis: Mosby.